GLIOBLASTOMA
AND HIGH GRADE GLIOMA

A guide for **managing your care**

DR. THOMAS GRUBER • MARCIA GRUBER-PAGE RN

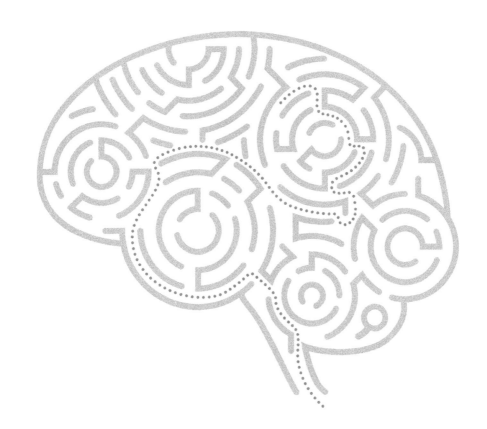

GLIOBLASTOMA
AND HIGH GRADE GLIOMA

A guide for managing your care

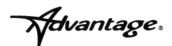

Published by Advantage, Charleston, South Carolina.
Member of Advantage Media Group.

ADVANTAGE is a registered trademark, and the Advantage colophon is a trademark of Advantage Media Group, Inc.

Printed in the United States of America.

10 9 8 7 6 5 4 3 2 1

ISBN: 978-1-64225-410-5
LCCN: 2022916799

Cover design by Analisa Smith.
Layout design by Wesley Strickland.

This publication is designed to provide accurate and authoritative information in regard to the subject matter covered. It is sold with the understanding that the publisher is not engaged in rendering legal, accounting, or other professional services. If legal advice or other expert assistance is required, the services of a competent professional person should be sought.

Advantage Media Group is a publisher of business, self-improvement, and professional development books and online learning. We help entrepreneurs, business leaders, and professionals share their Stories, Passion, and Knowledge to help others Learn & Grow. Do you have a manuscript or book idea that you would like us to consider for publishing? Please visit **advantagefamily.com**.

INTRODUCTION

When I walked past the exam room, I heard a sigh and a tearful sob. I entered the room and asked, "Can I help?" The patient sobbed, "It's too much. I'm scared. What if I forget something? Will I die?" Her husband asked, "How will we ever keep track of all of these appointments and all of her medications? I'm afraid of making a mistake; this is too important."

A gentleman knocked on my office door and asked if I had a three-hole punch that he could borrow. As I walked him over to the clerical station I asked what he needed it for. He pulled a three-ring binder out of his valise and said, "I'm keeping track of my son's test results, appointments, and disability papers for him," and he proudly showed me how he had created the index tabs so that he or his son could find the right sections.

I walked into the clinic reception area, and there was a woman on the floor picking up a stack of papers that she had dropped. I bent down to help her and realized these papers were copies of pathology reports, imaging reports, chemo schedules, a "cancer" diet article from the internet, insurance information, and various other information related to a patient's medical situation. She explained that the patient was her mother who was in the exam room with the doctor. She had dropped all the paperwork when she stood to accompany her mother into the exam room. I told her to go be with her mother and I would bring her all her papers. She asked if I could find a "big rubber band" so that she would not drop the papers again.

"You have cancer." These are the three most terrifying words in any language. They cause a tumult of emotions that range from fear and panic to denial and "why me?" to anger, anxiety, and depression. For most patients, they are so stunned by those words that their ability to hear and understand anything the doctor says after that is limited.

"Now what?" Several actions may be recommended by your doctor when you are first diagnosed and throughout treatment. Your doctor may recommend more diagnostic testing. Your doctor may talk with you about treatment options. Your doctor may refer you to a specialist or two or three.

"How do I remember all of this?" Cancer is a complicated disease, and so are the diagnostic and treatment processes. We have watched our patients and their families struggle to remember and keep track of the multiple appointments, procedures, specialists, test results, co-pays, sick leave, disability applications, and everything else that you take care of for your family and others who depend on you. As described in the real-life examples at the beginning of this introduction, we have seen patients and their families devise many ways to keep track of all the information—stacks of loose papers held together with rubber bands and clips, three-ring binders, black/white composition notebooks, two-ring binders with pockets, plastic supermarket bags, manilla folders, and various combinations of methods as an attempt by our patients and family to keep all their health-related information and reminders in order.

A diagnosis of any type of cancer is frightening, and the journey through diagnosis and treatment is complex and often confusing. A glioblastoma diagnosis can be particularly challenging, as the brain is the "control center" for our bodies. This book, *Glioblastoma and High Grade Glioma,* will walk you through the experience so that you know what to expect. This workbook, a guide for managing your care, is a companion to the book to help you track, manage, understand, and communicate the information that is important for you to progress through your medical care. The pages in the guide provide an easy way for you to list and organize your doctor and test appointments, treatment schedules, and dates of surgery and procedures. There is also a list of possible side effects for you to track and date, if they occur. "Notes" pages are included, and you can use these for anything you want—questions for the doctor or your innermost thoughts about your experience.

Another side effect of learning that you have cancer is the feeling that your life is spinning out of control and that the cancer is in charge. We created this book and guide to give you back some of that control.

This workbook is dedicated to my very first Nurse Manager, Mrs. Christine Robinson. Mrs. Robinson told me very early in my career that professional inspiration will come from our patients. She was right! The Guide for Managing Your Care *is dedicated to the countless number of courageous patients and their loved ones whom we have cared for during our respective careers. We have observed our patients struggle as they attempt to keep track of the copious amount of information related to their care and their diagnoses. It became clear to us that being able to organize and track their medical care is an important piece of regaining some control for our patients—and for the friends and family who are alongside the patient on this path. We designed this Guide to relieve some of the anxiety and give you back some control.*

PATIENT DEMOGRAPHICS

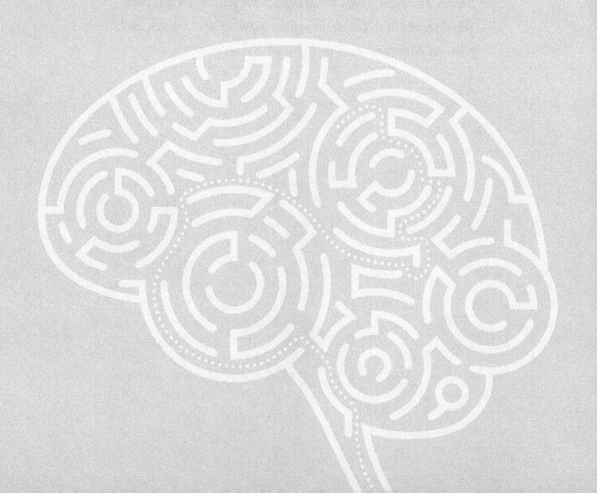

THIS BOOK BELONGS TO:

_____

_____

PHONE #: _____

IN CASE OF EMERGENCY:

_____

_____

PHONE #: _____

PRIMARY CARE DOCTOR:

_____

_____

PHONE #: _____

NEUROSURGEON:

_____

_____

PHONE #: _____

MEDICAL ONCOLOGIST:

_____

_____

PHONE #: _____

RADIATION ONCOLOGIST:

_____

_____

PHONE #: _____

OTHER DOCTOR(S):

PHONE #:

OTHER DOCTOR(S):

PHONE #:

NURSE NAVIGATOR:

PHONE #:

NURSE PRACTITIONER/PA:

PHONE #:

NURSE PRACTITIONER/PA:

PHONE #:

NURSE PRACTITIONER/PA:

PHONE #:

NOTES

NOTES

NOTES

INSURANCE AND PRESCRIPTION DRUG INFORMATION

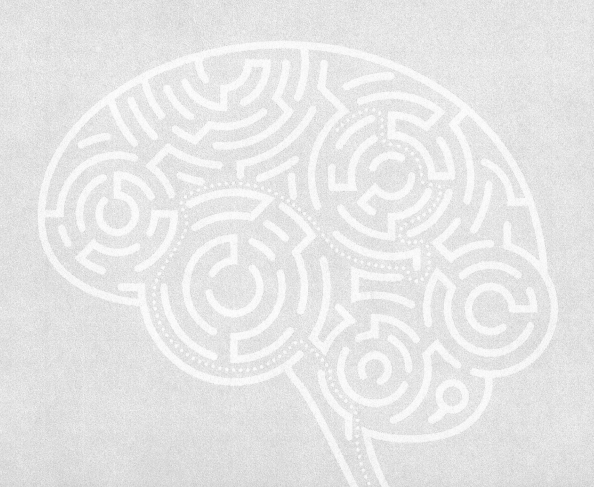

PRIMARY INSURANCE PROVIDER:

NAME OF POLICY HOLDER:

DOB OF PRIMARY POLICY HOLDER:

MEMBER ID #:   GROUP #:

PLAN TYPE: BENEFITS #:

SECONDARY INSURANCE PROVIDER:

NAME OF POLICY HOLDER:

DOB OF PRIMARY POLICY HOLDER:

MEMBER ID #:   GROUP #:

PLAN TYPE: BENEFITS #:

PRESCRIPTION DRUG ID CARD

PREFERRED PHARMACY:

ADDRESS:

ID #:

RxGRP:

RxBIN:

RxPCN:

PRESCRIPTION DRUG ID CARD

PREFERRED PHARMACY:

ADDRESS:

ID #:

RxGRP:

RxBIN:

RxPCN:

PRESCRIPTION MEDICATIONS:

DRUG NAME: DOSE:

HOW OFTEN?

REASON:

DOCTOR WHO PRESCRIBED:

DRUG NAME: DOSE:

HOW OFTEN?

REASON:

DOCTOR WHO PRESCRIBED:

DRUG NAME: DOSE:

HOW OFTEN?

REASON:

DOCTOR WHO PRESCRIBED:

DRUG NAME: DOSE:

HOW OFTEN?

REASON:

DOCTOR WHO PRESCRIBED:

PRESCRIPTION MEDICATIONS:

DRUG NAME: DOSE:

HOW OFTEN?

REASON:

DOCTOR WHO PRESCRIBED:

DRUG NAME: DOSE:

HOW OFTEN?

REASON:

DOCTOR WHO PRESCRIBED:

DRUG NAME: DOSE:

HOW OFTEN?

REASON:

DOCTOR WHO PRESCRIBED:

DRUG NAME: DOSE:

HOW OFTEN?

REASON:

DOCTOR WHO PRESCRIBED:

PRESCRIPTION MEDICATIONS:

DRUG NAME: DOSE:

HOW OFTEN?

REASON:

DOCTOR WHO PRESCRIBED:

DRUG NAME: DOSE:

HOW OFTEN?

REASON:

DOCTOR WHO PRESCRIBED:

DRUG NAME: DOSE:

HOW OFTEN?

REASON:

DOCTOR WHO PRESCRIBED:

DRUG NAME: DOSE:

HOW OFTEN?

REASON:

DOCTOR WHO PRESCRIBED:

PRESCRIPTION MEDICATIONS:

DRUG NAME: DOSE:

HOW OFTEN?

REASON:

DOCTOR WHO PRESCRIBED:

DRUG NAME: DOSE:

HOW OFTEN?

REASON:

DOCTOR WHO PRESCRIBED:

DRUG NAME: DOSE:

HOW OFTEN?

REASON:

DOCTOR WHO PRESCRIBED:

DRUG NAME: DOSE:

HOW OFTEN?

REASON:

DOCTOR WHO PRESCRIBED:

PRESCRIPTION MEDICATIONS:

DRUG NAME: DOSE:

HOW OFTEN?

REASON:

DOCTOR WHO PRESCRIBED:

DRUG NAME: DOSE:

HOW OFTEN?

REASON:

DOCTOR WHO PRESCRIBED:

DRUG NAME: DOSE:

HOW OFTEN?

REASON:

DOCTOR WHO PRESCRIBED:

DRUG NAME: DOSE:

HOW OFTEN?

REASON:

DOCTOR WHO PRESCRIBED:

OVER-THE-COUNTER MEDICATIONS, VITAMINS, AND HERBAL SUBSTANCES:

DRUG NAME: DOSE:

HOW OFTEN?

REASON:

DRUG NAME: DOSE:

HOW OFTEN?

REASON:

DRUG NAME: DOSE:

HOW OFTEN?

REASON:

DRUG NAME: DOSE:

HOW OFTEN?

REASON:

DRUG NAME: DOSE:

HOW OFTEN?

REASON:

OVER-THE-COUNTER MEDICATIONS, VITAMINS, AND HERBAL SUBSTANCES:

DRUG NAME: DOSE:

HOW OFTEN?

REASON:

DRUG NAME: DOSE:

HOW OFTEN?

REASON:

DRUG NAME: DOSE:

HOW OFTEN?

REASON:

DRUG NAME: DOSE:

HOW OFTEN?

REASON:

DRUG NAME: DOSE:

HOW OFTEN?

REASON:

NOTES

NOTES

SYMPTOM TRACKER

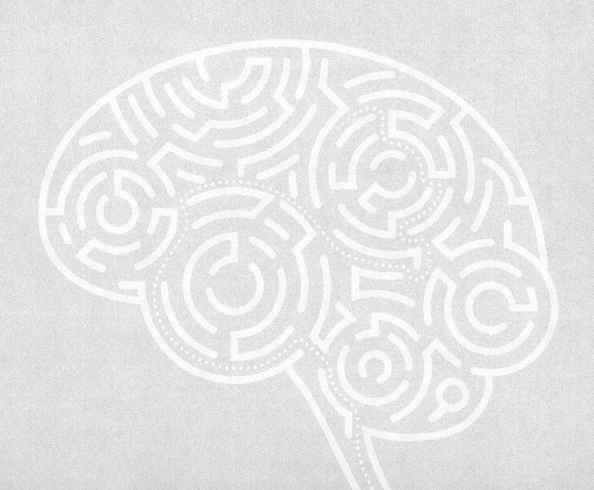

SYMPTOMS TO WATCH FOR AND REPORT TO YOUR DOCTOR:	DATE 1:	DATE 2:	DATE 3:	DATE 4:	DATE 5:
Difficulty sleeping					
Pain					
Appetite has changed					
I have an upset stomach, nausea or vomiting sometimes or often					
I have sores in my mouth or lips					
I am not able to do my normal daily activities					
I tire easily					
My vision has changed					
My hearing has changed					
My speech has changed or I'm slurring my words					
I am having difficulty finding the right words					
I am having difficulty thinking or feel confused sometimes					
I have headaches, more than usual					
I am forgetting things, my memory has changed					
Personality change – I am angry, sad or feel down at times for no reason					
I have abnormal movements in my arms or legs, seizures or convulsions					
Behavior change – no longer doing the normal daily activities					
I am having trouble walking					
I have weakness in arms or legs					
I sometimes lose my balance or have had a fall					
Fever					
Redness, swelling or drainage from surgical wound					

SYMPTOMS TO WATCH FOR AND REPORT TO YOUR DOCTOR:	DATE 1:	DATE 2:	DATE 3:	DATE 4:	DATE 5:
Difficulty sleeping					
Pain					
Appetite has changed					
I have an upset stomach, nausea or vomiting sometimes or often					
I have sores in my mouth or lips					
I am not able to do my normal daily activities					
I tire easily					
My vision has changed					
My hearing has changed					
My speech has changed or I'm slurring my words					
I am having difficulty finding the right words					
I am having difficulty thinking or feel confused sometimes					
I have headaches, more than usual					
I am forgetting things, my memory has changed					
Personality change - I am angry, sad or feel down at times for no reason					
I have abnormal movements in my arms or legs, seizures or convulsions					
Behavior change - no longer doing the normal daily activities					
I am having trouble walking					
I have weakness in arms or legs					
I sometimes lose my balance or have had a fall					
Fever					
Redness, swelling or drainage from surgical wound					

SYMPTOMS TO WATCH FOR AND REPORT TO YOUR DOCTOR:	DATE 1:	DATE 2:	DATE 3:	DATE 4:	DATE 5:

NOTES

NOTES

PATIENT SURGERY

NEUROSURGEON CONTACT INFORMATION

NAME OF DOCTOR:

NAME OF NP OR PA:

NURSE/NURSE NAVIGATOR:

SCHEDULER:

NAME OF PRACTICE:

ADDRESS:

PHONE NUMBER:

PATIENT PORTAL:

ADDITIONAL INFO:

SURGERY LOG

TYPE OF SURGERY:

☐ BIOPSY ONLY   ☐ CRANIOTOMY

☐ GLIADEL WAFER PLACEMENT   ☐ GAMMA TILE PLACEMENT

☐ LASER INTERSTITIAL TREATMENT   ☐ OTHER:

DATE OF SURGERY:

SURGEON NAME:

LOCATION OF SURGERY:

DISCHARGE DATE:

ADDITIONAL INFO:

SURGERY LOG

TYPE OF SURGERY:

- ☐ BIOPSY ONLY
- ☐ CRANIOTOMY
- ☐ GLIADEL WAFER PLACEMENT
- ☐ GAMMA TILE PLACEMENT
- ☐ LASER INTERSTITIAL TREATMENT
- ☐ OTHER:

DATE OF SURGERY:

SURGEON NAME:

LOCATION OF SURGERY:

DISCHARGE DATE:

ADDITIONAL INFO:

SURGERY LOG

TYPE OF SURGERY:

☐ BIOPSY ONLY   ☐ CRANIOTOMY

☐ GLIADEL WAFER PLACEMENT   ☐ GAMMA TILE PLACEMENT

☐ LASER INTERSTITIAL TREATMENT   ☐ OTHER:

DATE OF SURGERY:

SURGEON NAME:

LOCATION OF SURGERY:

DISCHARGE DATE:

ADDITIONAL INFO:

SURGERY LOG

TYPE OF SURGERY:

☐ BIOPSY ONLY   ☐ CRANIOTOMY

☐ GLIADEL WAFER PLACEMENT   ☐ GAMMA TILE PLACEMENT

☐ LASER INTERSTITIAL TREATMENT   ☐ OTHER:

DATE OF SURGERY:

SURGEON NAME:

LOCATION OF SURGERY:

DISCHARGE DATE:

ADDITIONAL INFO:

NOTES

NOTES

NEUROSURGERY APPOINTMENT

NEUROSURGEON SUMMARY
OF CLINIC APPOINTMENT

DATE:

DOCTOR SEEN:

☐ PRE SURGERY EVALUATION   ☐ POST SURGERY FOLLOWUP

☐ OTHER (SPECIFY):

TESTING DONE:

QUESTIONS FOR DOCTOR/PRACTITIONER:

SUMMARY OF VISIT

RESULTS OF TESTING:

TESTING ORDERED FOR NEXT VISIT:

MEDICATION CHANGES:

REFERRALS:

NEUROSURGEON SUMMARY OF CLINIC APPOINTMENT

DATE:

DOCTOR SEEN:

☐ PRE SURGERY EVALUATION   ☐ POST SURGERY FOLLOWUP

☐ OTHER (SPECIFY):

TESTING DONE:

QUESTIONS FOR DOCTOR/PRACTITIONER:

SUMMARY OF VISIT

RESULTS OF TESTING:

TESTING ORDERED FOR NEXT VISIT:

MEDICATION CHANGES:

REFERRALS:

NEUROSURGEON SUMMARY
OF CLINIC APPOINTMENT

DATE:
_____

DOCTOR SEEN:
_____

☐ PRE SURGERY EVALUATION   ☐ POST SURGERY FOLLOWUP

☐ OTHER (SPECIFY):

TESTING DONE:

QUESTIONS FOR DOCTOR/PRACTITIONER:
_____
_____
_____
_____

SUMMARY OF VISIT

RESULTS OF TESTING:
_____
_____

TESTING ORDERED FOR NEXT VISIT:
_____
_____

MEDICATION CHANGES:
_____
_____

REFERRALS:
_____

NEUROSURGEON SUMMARY OF CLINIC APPOINTMENT

DATE:

DOCTOR SEEN:

☐ PRE SURGERY EVALUATION   ☐ POST SURGERY FOLLOWUP

☐ OTHER (SPECIFY):

TESTING DONE:

QUESTIONS FOR DOCTOR/PRACTITIONER:

SUMMARY OF VISIT

RESULTS OF TESTING:

TESTING ORDERED FOR NEXT VISIT:

MEDICATION CHANGES:

REFERRALS:

NEUROSURGEON SUMMARY
OF CLINIC APPOINTMENT

DATE:

DOCTOR SEEN:

☐ PRE SURGERY EVALUATION   ☐ POST SURGERY FOLLOWUP

☐ OTHER (SPECIFY):

TESTING DONE:

QUESTIONS FOR DOCTOR/PRACTITIONER:

SUMMARY OF VISIT

RESULTS OF TESTING:

TESTING ORDERED FOR NEXT VISIT:

MEDICATION CHANGES:

REFERRALS:

NEUROSURGEON SUMMARY OF CLINIC APPOINTMENT

DATE:

DOCTOR SEEN:

☐ PRE SURGERY EVALUATION   ☐ POST SURGERY FOLLOWUP

☐ OTHER (SPECIFY):

TESTING DONE:

QUESTIONS FOR DOCTOR/PRACTITIONER:

SUMMARY OF VISIT

RESULTS OF TESTING:

TESTING ORDERED FOR NEXT VISIT:

MEDICATION CHANGES:

REFERRALS:

NEUROSURGEON SUMMARY
OF CLINIC APPOINTMENT

DATE:

DOCTOR SEEN:

☐ PRE SURGERY EVALUATION   ☐ POST SURGERY FOLLOWUP

☐ OTHER (SPECIFY):

TESTING DONE:

QUESTIONS FOR DOCTOR/PRACTITIONER:

SUMMARY OF VISIT

RESULTS OF TESTING:

TESTING ORDERED FOR NEXT VISIT:

MEDICATION CHANGES:

REFERRALS:

NEUROSURGEON SUMMARY OF CLINIC APPOINTMENT

DATE:

DOCTOR SEEN:

☐ PRE SURGERY EVALUATION ☐ POST SURGERY FOLLOWUP

☐ OTHER (SPECIFY):

TESTING DONE:

QUESTIONS FOR DOCTOR/PRACTITIONER:

SUMMARY OF VISIT

RESULTS OF TESTING:

TESTING ORDERED FOR NEXT VISIT:

MEDICATION CHANGES:

REFERRALS:

NEUROSURGEON SUMMARY
OF CLINIC APPOINTMENT

DATE:

DOCTOR SEEN:

☐ PRE SURGERY EVALUATION   ☐ POST SURGERY FOLLOWUP

☐ OTHER (SPECIFY):

TESTING DONE:

QUESTIONS FOR DOCTOR/PRACTITIONER:

SUMMARY OF VISIT

RESULTS OF TESTING:

TESTING ORDERED FOR NEXT VISIT:

MEDICATION CHANGES:

REFERRALS:

NEUROSURGEON SUMMARY OF CLINIC APPOINTMENT

DATE:

DOCTOR SEEN:

☐ PRE SURGERY EVALUATION   ☐ POST SURGERY FOLLOWUP

☐ OTHER (SPECIFY):

TESTING DONE:

QUESTIONS FOR DOCTOR/PRACTITIONER:

SUMMARY OF VISIT

RESULTS OF TESTING:

TESTING ORDERED FOR NEXT VISIT:

MEDICATION CHANGES:

REFERRALS:

NEUROSURGEON SUMMARY
OF CLINIC APPOINTMENT

DATE:
_____

DOCTOR SEEN:
_____

☐ PRE SURGERY EVALUATION ☐ POST SURGERY FOLLOWUP

☐ OTHER (SPECIFY):
_____

TESTING DONE:
_____

QUESTIONS FOR DOCTOR/PRACTITIONER:
_____
_____
_____
_____

SUMMARY OF VISIT

RESULTS OF TESTING:
_____
_____

TESTING ORDERED FOR NEXT VISIT:
_____
_____

MEDICATION CHANGES:
_____
_____

REFERRALS:
_____

NEUROSURGEON SUMMARY
OF CLINIC APPOINTMENT

DATE:

DOCTOR SEEN:

☐ PRE SURGERY EVALUATION   ☐ POST SURGERY FOLLOWUP

☐ OTHER (SPECIFY):

TESTING DONE:

QUESTIONS FOR DOCTOR/PRACTITIONER:

SUMMARY OF VISIT

RESULTS OF TESTING:

TESTING ORDERED FOR NEXT VISIT:

MEDICATION CHANGES:

REFERRALS:

NOTES

RADIATION ONCOLOGY

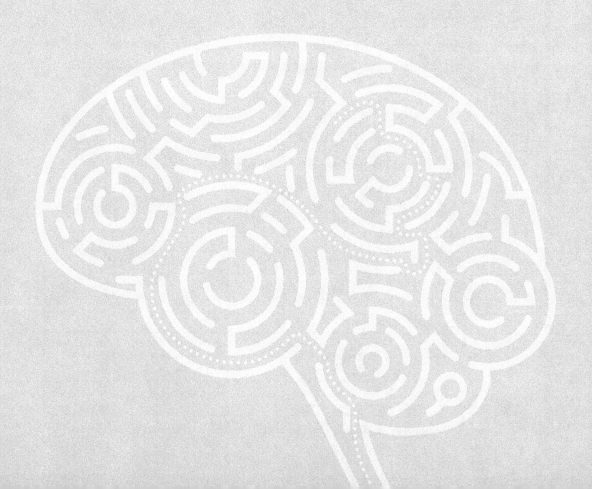

RADIATION ONCOLOGIST CONTACT INFORMATION

NAME OF DOCTOR:

NAME OF NP OR PA:

NURSE/NURSE NAVIGATOR:

SCHEDULER:

NAME OF PRACTICE:

ADDRESS:

PHONE NUMBER:

PATIENT PORTAL:

ADDITIONAL INFO:

RADIATION ONCOLOGY LOG

☐ STEREOTACTIC RADIATION (SRS)

☐ INTENSITY MODULATED RADIATION THERAPY (IMRT)

☐ OTHER (SPECIFY):

NUMBER OF TREATMENTS PLANNED:

NUMBER OF TREATMENTS RECEIVED:

START DATE:

END DATE:

SIDE EFFECTS:

RADIATION ONCOLOGY LOG

☐ STEREOTACTIC RADIATION (SRS)

☐ INTENSITY MODULATED RADIATION THERAPY (IMRT)

☐ OTHER (SPECIFY):

NUMBER OF TREATMENTS PLANNED:

NUMBER OF TREATMENTS RECEIVED:

START DATE:

END DATE:

SIDE EFFECTS:

RADIATION ONCOLOGY LOG

☐ STEREOTACTIC RADIATION (SRS)

☐ INTENSITY MODULATED RADIATION THERAPY (IMRT)

☐ OTHER (SPECIFY):

NUMBER OF TREATMENTS PLANNED:

NUMBER OF TREATMENTS RECEIVED:

START DATE:

END DATE:

SIDE EFFECTS:

NOTES

RADIATION ONCOLOGY APPOINTMENT

RADIATION ONCOLOGY SUMMARY
OF CLINIC APPOINTMENT

DATE:

DOCTOR SEEN:

☐ PRETREATMENT EVALUATION   ☐ POST TREATMENT FOLLOWUP

☐ OTHER:

TESTING DONE:

QUESTIONS FOR DOCTOR/PRACTITIONER:

SUMMARY OF VISIT

RESULTS OF TESTING:

TESTING ORDERED FOR NEXT VISIT:

MEDICATION CHANGES:

REFERRALS:

RADIATION ONCOLOGY SUMMARY OF CLINIC APPOINTMENT

DATE:

DOCTOR SEEN:

☐ PRETREATMENT EVALUATION   ☐ POST TREATMENT FOLLOWUP

☐ OTHER:

TESTING DONE:

QUESTIONS FOR DOCTOR/PRACTITIONER:

SUMMARY OF VISIT

RESULTS OF TESTING:

TESTING ORDERED FOR NEXT VISIT:

MEDICATION CHANGES:

REFERRALS:

RADIATION ONCOLOGY SUMMARY OF CLINIC APPOINTMENT

DATE:

_____

DOCTOR SEEN:

_____

☐ PRETREATMENT EVALUATION   ☐ POST TREATMENT FOLLOWUP

☐ OTHER:

_____

TESTING DONE:

_____

QUESTIONS FOR DOCTOR/PRACTITIONER:

_____

_____

_____

_____

SUMMARY OF VISIT

RESULTS OF TESTING:

_____

_____

TESTING ORDERED FOR NEXT VISIT:

_____

_____

MEDICATION CHANGES:

_____

_____

REFERRALS:

_____

RADIATION ONCOLOGY SUMMARY OF CLINIC APPOINTMENT

DATE:

DOCTOR SEEN:

☐ PRETREATMENT EVALUATION ☐ POST TREATMENT FOLLOWUP

☐ OTHER:

TESTING DONE:

QUESTIONS FOR DOCTOR/PRACTITIONER:

SUMMARY OF VISIT

RESULTS OF TESTING:

TESTING ORDERED FOR NEXT VISIT:

MEDICATION CHANGES:

REFERRALS:

RADIATION ONCOLOGY SUMMARY
OF CLINIC APPOINTMENT

DATE:

DOCTOR SEEN:

☐ PRETREATMENT EVALUATION   ☐ POST TREATMENT FOLLOWUP

☐ OTHER:

TESTING DONE:

QUESTIONS FOR DOCTOR/PRACTITIONER:

SUMMARY OF VISIT

RESULTS OF TESTING:

TESTING ORDERED FOR NEXT VISIT:

MEDICATION CHANGES:

REFERRALS:

RADIATION ONCOLOGY SUMMARY OF CLINIC APPOINTMENT

DATE:

DOCTOR SEEN:

☐ PRETREATMENT EVALUATION   ☐ POST TREATMENT FOLLOWUP

☐ OTHER:

TESTING DONE:

QUESTIONS FOR DOCTOR/PRACTITIONER:

SUMMARY OF VISIT

RESULTS OF TESTING:

TESTING ORDERED FOR NEXT VISIT:

MEDICATION CHANGES:

REFERRALS:

RADIATION ONCOLOGY SUMMARY OF CLINIC APPOINTMENT

DATE:

DOCTOR SEEN:

☐ PRETREATMENT EVALUATION   ☐ POST TREATMENT FOLLOWUP

☐ OTHER:

TESTING DONE:

QUESTIONS FOR DOCTOR/PRACTITIONER:

SUMMARY OF VISIT

RESULTS OF TESTING:

TESTING ORDERED FOR NEXT VISIT:

MEDICATION CHANGES:

REFERRALS:

RADIATION ONCOLOGY SUMMARY OF CLINIC APPOINTMENT

DATE:

DOCTOR SEEN:

☐ PRETREATMENT EVALUATION   ☐ POST TREATMENT FOLLOWUP

☐ OTHER:

TESTING DONE:

QUESTIONS FOR DOCTOR/PRACTITIONER:

SUMMARY OF VISIT

RESULTS OF TESTING:

TESTING ORDERED FOR NEXT VISIT:

MEDICATION CHANGES:

REFERRALS:

RADIATION ONCOLOGY SUMMARY
OF CLINIC APPOINTMENT

DATE:

DOCTOR SEEN:

☐ PRETREATMENT EVALUATION   ☐ POST TREATMENT FOLLOWUP

☐ OTHER:

TESTING DONE:

QUESTIONS FOR DOCTOR/PRACTITIONER:

SUMMARY OF VISIT

RESULTS OF TESTING:

TESTING ORDERED FOR NEXT VISIT:

MEDICATION CHANGES:

REFERRALS:

RADIATION ONCOLOGY SUMMARY OF CLINIC APPOINTMENT

DATE:

DOCTOR SEEN:

☐ PRETREATMENT EVALUATION   ☐ POST TREATMENT FOLLOWUP

☐ OTHER:

TESTING DONE:

QUESTIONS FOR DOCTOR/PRACTITIONER:

SUMMARY OF VISIT

RESULTS OF TESTING:

TESTING ORDERED FOR NEXT VISIT:

MEDICATION CHANGES:

REFERRALS:

RADIATION ONCOLOGY SUMMARY OF CLINIC APPOINTMENT

DATE:

DOCTOR SEEN:

☐ PRETREATMENT EVALUATION   ☐ POST TREATMENT FOLLOWUP

☐ OTHER:

TESTING DONE:

QUESTIONS FOR DOCTOR/PRACTITIONER:

SUMMARY OF VISIT

RESULTS OF TESTING:

TESTING ORDERED FOR NEXT VISIT:

MEDICATION CHANGES:

REFERRALS:

RADIATION ONCOLOGY SUMMARY OF CLINIC APPOINTMENT

DATE:

DOCTOR SEEN:

☐ PRETREATMENT EVALUATION ☐ POST TREATMENT FOLLOWUP

☐ OTHER:

TESTING DONE:

QUESTIONS FOR DOCTOR/PRACTITIONER:

SUMMARY OF VISIT

RESULTS OF TESTING:

TESTING ORDERED FOR NEXT VISIT:

MEDICATION CHANGES:

REFERRALS:

NOTES

MEDICAL ONCOLOGY

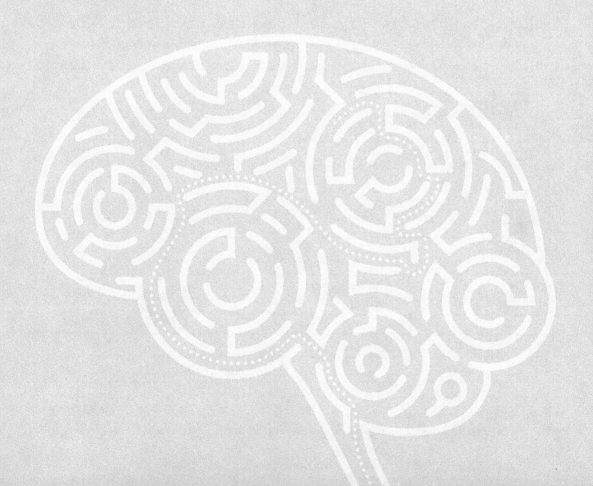

MEDICAL ONCOLOGY
CONTACT INFORMATION

NAME OF DOCTOR:

NAME OF NP OR PA:

NURSE/NURSE NAVIGATOR:

SCHEDULER:

NAME OF PRACTICE:

ADDRESS:

PHONE NUMBER:

PATIENT PORTAL:

ADDITIONAL INFO:

MEDICAL ONCOLOGY SUMMARY OF CLINIC APPOINTMENT

DATE:

DOCTOR SEEN:

☐ NEW PATIENT VISIT   ☐ ROUTINE FOLLOWUP

☐ URGENT CARE VISIT   ☐ OTHER:

TESTING DONE:

QUESTIONS FOR DOCTOR/PRACTITIONER:

SUMMARY OF VISIT

RESULTS OF TESTING:

TESTING ORDERED FOR NEXT VISIT:

MEDICATION CHANGES:

REFERRALS:

MEDICAL ONCOLOGY SUMMARY OF CLINIC APPOINTMENT

DATE:

DOCTOR SEEN:

☐ NEW PATIENT VISIT   ☐ ROUTINE FOLLOWUP

☐ URGENT CARE VISIT   ☐ OTHER:

TESTING DONE:

QUESTIONS FOR DOCTOR/PRACTITIONER:

SUMMARY OF VISIT

RESULTS OF TESTING:

TESTING ORDERED FOR NEXT VISIT:

MEDICATION CHANGES:

REFERRALS:

MEDICAL ONCOLOGY SUMMARY OF CLINIC APPOINTMENT

DATE:
_____

DOCTOR SEEN:
_____

☐ NEW PATIENT VISIT   ☐ ROUTINE FOLLOWUP

☐ URGENT CARE VISIT   ☐ OTHER:

TESTING DONE:
_____

QUESTIONS FOR DOCTOR/PRACTITIONER:
_____
_____
_____
_____

SUMMARY OF VISIT

RESULTS OF TESTING:
_____
_____

TESTING ORDERED FOR NEXT VISIT:
_____
_____

MEDICATION CHANGES:
_____
_____

REFERRALS:
_____

MEDICAL ONCOLOGY SUMMARY OF CLINIC APPOINTMENT

DATE:

DOCTOR SEEN:

☐ NEW PATIENT VISIT   ☐ ROUTINE FOLLOWUP

☐ URGENT CARE VISIT   ☐ OTHER:

TESTING DONE:

QUESTIONS FOR DOCTOR/PRACTITIONER:

SUMMARY OF VISIT

RESULTS OF TESTING:

TESTING ORDERED FOR NEXT VISIT:

MEDICATION CHANGES:

REFERRALS:

MEDICAL ONCOLOGY SUMMARY OF CLINIC APPOINTMENT

DATE:

DOCTOR SEEN:

☐ NEW PATIENT VISIT   ☐ ROUTINE FOLLOWUP

☐ URGENT CARE VISIT   ☐ OTHER:

TESTING DONE:

QUESTIONS FOR DOCTOR/PRACTITIONER:

SUMMARY OF VISIT

RESULTS OF TESTING:

TESTING ORDERED FOR NEXT VISIT:

MEDICATION CHANGES:

REFERRALS:

MEDICAL ONCOLOGY SUMMARY OF CLINIC APPOINTMENT

DATE:

DOCTOR SEEN:

☐ NEW PATIENT VISIT   ☐ ROUTINE FOLLOWUP

☐ URGENT CARE VISIT   ☐ OTHER:

TESTING DONE:

QUESTIONS FOR DOCTOR/PRACTITIONER:

SUMMARY OF VISIT

RESULTS OF TESTING:

TESTING ORDERED FOR NEXT VISIT:

MEDICATION CHANGES:

REFERRALS:

MEDICAL ONCOLOGY SUMMARY OF CLINIC APPOINTMENT

DATE:
_____

DOCTOR SEEN:
_____

☐ NEW PATIENT VISIT ☐ ROUTINE FOLLOWUP

☐ URGENT CARE VISIT ☐ OTHER:
_____

TESTING DONE:
_____

QUESTIONS FOR DOCTOR/PRACTITIONER:
_____
_____
_____
_____
_____

SUMMARY OF VISIT

RESULTS OF TESTING:
_____
_____

TESTING ORDERED FOR NEXT VISIT:
_____
_____

MEDICATION CHANGES:
_____
_____

REFERRALS:
_____

MEDICAL ONCOLOGY SUMMARY OF CLINIC APPOINTMENT

DATE:

DOCTOR SEEN:

☐ NEW PATIENT VISIT   ☐ ROUTINE FOLLOWUP

☐ URGENT CARE VISIT   ☐ OTHER:

TESTING DONE:

QUESTIONS FOR DOCTOR/PRACTITIONER:

SUMMARY OF VISIT

RESULTS OF TESTING:

TESTING ORDERED FOR NEXT VISIT:

MEDICATION CHANGES:

REFERRALS:

MEDICAL ONCOLOGY SUMMARY OF CLINIC APPOINTMENT

DATE:
_____

DOCTOR SEEN:
_____

☐ NEW PATIENT VISIT   ☐ ROUTINE FOLLOWUP

☐ URGENT CARE VISIT   ☐ OTHER:

TESTING DONE:
_____

QUESTIONS FOR DOCTOR/PRACTITIONER:
_____
_____
_____
_____

SUMMARY OF VISIT

RESULTS OF TESTING:
_____
_____

TESTING ORDERED FOR NEXT VISIT:
_____
_____

MEDICATION CHANGES:
_____
_____

REFERRALS:
_____

MEDICAL ONCOLOGY SUMMARY OF CLINIC APPOINTMENT

DATE:

DOCTOR SEEN:

☐ NEW PATIENT VISIT   ☐ ROUTINE FOLLOWUP

☐ URGENT CARE VISIT   ☐ OTHER:

TESTING DONE:

QUESTIONS FOR DOCTOR/PRACTITIONER:

SUMMARY OF VISIT

RESULTS OF TESTING:

TESTING ORDERED FOR NEXT VISIT:

MEDICATION CHANGES:

REFERRALS:

MEDICAL ONCOLOGY SUMMARY OF CLINIC APPOINTMENT

DATE:

DOCTOR SEEN:

☐ NEW PATIENT VISIT ☐ ROUTINE FOLLOWUP

☐ URGENT CARE VISIT ☐ OTHER:

TESTING DONE:

QUESTIONS FOR DOCTOR/PRACTITIONER:

SUMMARY OF VISIT

RESULTS OF TESTING:

TESTING ORDERED FOR NEXT VISIT:

MEDICATION CHANGES:

REFERRALS:

MEDICAL ONCOLOGY SUMMARY
OF CLINIC APPOINTMENT

DATE:
_____

DOCTOR SEEN:
_____

☐ NEW PATIENT VISIT   ☐ ROUTINE FOLLOWUP

☐ URGENT CARE VISIT   ☐ OTHER:
_____

TESTING DONE:

QUESTIONS FOR DOCTOR/PRACTITIONER:
_____
_____
_____
_____

SUMMARY OF VISIT

RESULTS OF TESTING:
_____
_____

TESTING ORDERED FOR NEXT VISIT:
_____
_____

MEDICATION CHANGES:
_____
_____

REFERRALS:
_____

MEDICAL ONCOLOGY SUMMARY OF CLINIC APPOINTMENT

DATE:

DOCTOR SEEN:

☐ NEW PATIENT VISIT   ☐ ROUTINE FOLLOWUP

☐ URGENT CARE VISIT   ☐ OTHER:

TESTING DONE:

QUESTIONS FOR DOCTOR/PRACTITIONER:

SUMMARY OF VISIT

RESULTS OF TESTING:

TESTING ORDERED FOR NEXT VISIT:

MEDICATION CHANGES:

REFERRALS:

MEDICAL ONCOLOGY SUMMARY
OF CLINIC APPOINTMENT

DATE:
_____

DOCTOR SEEN:
_____

☐ NEW PATIENT VISIT   ☐ ROUTINE FOLLOWUP

☐ URGENT CARE VISIT   ☐ OTHER:

TESTING DONE:
_____

QUESTIONS FOR DOCTOR/PRACTITIONER:
_____
_____
_____
_____
_____

SUMMARY OF VISIT

RESULTS OF TESTING:
_____
_____

TESTING ORDERED FOR NEXT VISIT:
_____
_____

MEDICATION CHANGES:
_____
_____

REFERRALS:
_____

MEDICAL ONCOLOGY SUMMARY OF CLINIC APPOINTMENT

DATE:

DOCTOR SEEN:

☐ NEW PATIENT VISIT   ☐ ROUTINE FOLLOWUP

☐ URGENT CARE VISIT   ☐ OTHER:

TESTING DONE:

QUESTIONS FOR DOCTOR/PRACTITIONER:

SUMMARY OF VISIT

RESULTS OF TESTING:

TESTING ORDERED FOR NEXT VISIT:

MEDICATION CHANGES:

REFERRALS:

MEDICAL ONCOLOGY SUMMARY
OF CLINIC APPOINTMENT

DATE:

DOCTOR SEEN:

☐ NEW PATIENT VISIT   ☐ ROUTINE FOLLOWUP

☐ URGENT CARE VISIT   ☐ OTHER:

TESTING DONE:

QUESTIONS FOR DOCTOR/PRACTITIONER:

SUMMARY OF VISIT

RESULTS OF TESTING:

TESTING ORDERED FOR NEXT VISIT:

MEDICATION CHANGES:

REFERRALS:

MEDICAL ONCOLOGY SUMMARY
OF CLINIC APPOINTMENT

DATE:

DOCTOR SEEN:

☐ NEW PATIENT VISIT   ☐ ROUTINE FOLLOWUP

☐ URGENT CARE VISIT   ☐ OTHER:

TESTING DONE:

QUESTIONS FOR DOCTOR/PRACTITIONER:

SUMMARY OF VISIT

RESULTS OF TESTING:

TESTING ORDERED FOR NEXT VISIT:

MEDICATION CHANGES:

REFERRALS:

MEDICAL ONCOLOGY SUMMARY OF CLINIC APPOINTMENT

DATE:

DOCTOR SEEN:

☐ NEW PATIENT VISIT ☐ ROUTINE FOLLOWUP

☐ URGENT CARE VISIT ☐ OTHER:

TESTING DONE:

QUESTIONS FOR DOCTOR/PRACTITIONER:

SUMMARY OF VISIT

RESULTS OF TESTING:

TESTING ORDERED FOR NEXT VISIT:

MEDICATION CHANGES:

REFERRALS:

MEDICAL ONCOLOGY SUMMARY OF CLINIC APPOINTMENT

DATE:

DOCTOR SEEN:

☐ NEW PATIENT VISIT   ☐ ROUTINE FOLLOWUP

☐ URGENT CARE VISIT   ☐ OTHER:

TESTING DONE:

QUESTIONS FOR DOCTOR/PRACTITIONER:

SUMMARY OF VISIT

RESULTS OF TESTING:

TESTING ORDERED FOR NEXT VISIT:

MEDICATION CHANGES:

REFERRALS:

MEDICAL ONCOLOGY SUMMARY
OF CLINIC APPOINTMENT

DATE:

_____

DOCTOR SEEN:

_____

☐ NEW PATIENT VISIT   ☐ ROUTINE FOLLOWUP

☐ URGENT CARE VISIT   ☐ OTHER:

TESTING DONE:

_____

QUESTIONS FOR DOCTOR/PRACTITIONER:

_____

_____

_____

_____

SUMMARY OF VISIT

RESULTS OF TESTING:

_____

_____

TESTING ORDERED FOR NEXT VISIT:

_____

_____

MEDICATION CHANGES:

_____

_____

REFERRALS:

_____

MEDICAL ONCOLOGY SUMMARY OF CLINIC APPOINTMENT

DATE:

DOCTOR SEEN:

☐ NEW PATIENT VISIT   ☐ ROUTINE FOLLOWUP

☐ URGENT CARE VISIT   ☐ OTHER:

TESTING DONE:

QUESTIONS FOR DOCTOR/PRACTITIONER:

SUMMARY OF VISIT

RESULTS OF TESTING:

TESTING ORDERED FOR NEXT VISIT:

MEDICATION CHANGES:

REFERRALS:

MEDICAL ONCOLOGY SUMMARY OF CLINIC APPOINTMENT

DATE:
_____

DOCTOR SEEN:
_____

☐ NEW PATIENT VISIT   ☐ ROUTINE FOLLOWUP

☐ URGENT CARE VISIT   ☐ OTHER:

TESTING DONE:
_____

QUESTIONS FOR DOCTOR/PRACTITIONER:
_____
_____
_____
_____

SUMMARY OF VISIT

RESULTS OF TESTING:
_____
_____

TESTING ORDERED FOR NEXT VISIT:
_____
_____

MEDICATION CHANGES:
_____
_____

REFERRALS:
_____

MEDICAL ONCOLOGY SUMMARY OF CLINIC APPOINTMENT

DATE:

DOCTOR SEEN:

☐ NEW PATIENT VISIT   ☐ ROUTINE FOLLOWUP

☐ URGENT CARE VISIT   ☐ OTHER:

TESTING DONE:

QUESTIONS FOR DOCTOR/PRACTITIONER:

SUMMARY OF VISIT

RESULTS OF TESTING:

TESTING ORDERED FOR NEXT VISIT:

MEDICATION CHANGES:

REFERRALS:

MEDICAL ONCOLOGY SUMMARY OF CLINIC APPOINTMENT

DATE:

DOCTOR SEEN:

☐ NEW PATIENT VISIT   ☐ ROUTINE FOLLOWUP

☐ URGENT CARE VISIT   ☐ OTHER:

TESTING DONE:

QUESTIONS FOR DOCTOR/PRACTITIONER:

SUMMARY OF VISIT

RESULTS OF TESTING:

TESTING ORDERED FOR NEXT VISIT:

MEDICATION CHANGES:

REFERRALS:

MEDICAL ONCOLOGY SUMMARY OF CLINIC APPOINTMENT

DATE:

DOCTOR SEEN:

☐ NEW PATIENT VISIT   ☐ ROUTINE FOLLOWUP

☐ URGENT CARE VISIT   ☐ OTHER:

TESTING DONE:

QUESTIONS FOR DOCTOR/PRACTITIONER:

SUMMARY OF VISIT

RESULTS OF TESTING:

TESTING ORDERED FOR NEXT VISIT:

MEDICATION CHANGES:

REFERRALS:

NOTES

NOTES

NOTES

MEDICATION LOG
AND SCHEDULE

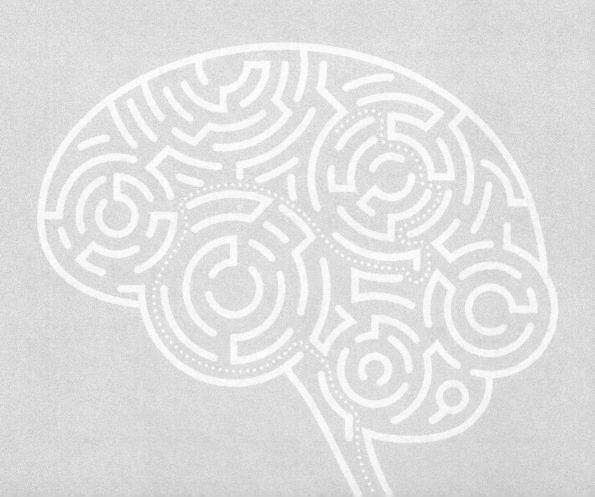

TEMODAR LOG

START DATE OF INITIAL CYCLE DURING RADIATION:
_____

END DATE OF INITIAL CYCLE DURING RADIATION:
_____

DOSE:
_____

NOTES:
_____
_____

START DATE 5 DAY CYCLE:
_____

DOSE:
_____

NOTES:
_____
_____

START DATE 5 DAY CYCLE:
_____

DOSE:
_____

NOTES:
_____
_____

START DATE 5 DAY CYCLE:
_____

DOSE:
_____

NOTES:
_____
_____
_____

START DATE 5 DAY CYCLE:

DOSE:

NOTES:

START DATE 5 DAY CYCLE:

DOSE:

NOTES:

START DATE 5 DAY CYCLE:

DOSE:

NOTES:

START DATE 5 DAY CYCLE:

DOSE:

NOTES:

START DATE 5 DAY CYCLE:

DOSE:

NOTES:

START DATE 5 DAY CYCLE:

DOSE:

NOTES:

START DATE 5 DAY CYCLE:

DOSE:

NOTES:

START DATE 5 DAY CYCLE:

DOSE:

NOTES:

START DATE 5 DAY CYCLE:
_____

DOSE:
_____

NOTES:
_____
_____
_____

START DATE 5 DAY CYCLE:
_____

DOSE:
_____

NOTES:
_____
_____
_____

START DATE 5 DAY CYCLE:
_____

DOSE:
_____

NOTES:
_____
_____
_____

START DATE 5 DAY CYCLE:
_____

DOSE:
_____

NOTES:
_____
_____

DECADRON LOG

START DATE:

END DATE:

REASON FOR DECADRON:

☐ RADIATION TREATMENT ☐ BRAIN SWELLING

☐ SURGERY ☐ OTHER

NOTES:

START DATE:

END DATE:

REASON FOR DECADRON:

☐ RADIATION TREATMENT ☐ BRAIN SWELLING

☐ SURGERY ☐ OTHER

NOTES:

START DATE:

END DATE:

REASON FOR DECADRON:

☐ RADIATION TREATMENT   ☐ BRAIN SWELLING

☐ SURGERY   ☐ OTHER

NOTES:

START DATE:

END DATE:

REASON FOR DECADRON:

☐ RADIATION TREATMENT   ☐ BRAIN SWELLING

☐ SURGERY   ☐ OTHER

NOTES:

START DATE:

END DATE:

REASON FOR DECADRON:

☐ RADIATION TREATMENT   ☐ BRAIN SWELLING

☐ SURGERY   ☐ OTHER

NOTES:

START DATE:

END DATE:

REASON FOR DECADRON:

☐ RADIATION TREATMENT   ☐ BRAIN SWELLING

☐ SURGERY   ☐ OTHER

NOTES:

START DATE:

END DATE:

REASON FOR DECADRON:

☐ RADIATION TREATMENT   ☐ BRAIN SWELLING

☐ SURGERY   ☐ OTHER

NOTES:

START DATE:

END DATE:

REASON FOR DECADRON:

☐ RADIATION TREATMENT   ☐ BRAIN SWELLING

☐ SURGERY   ☐ OTHER

NOTES:

ANTI-SEIZURE MEDICATION LOG

NAME OF MEDICATION: _____

☐ KEPPRA ☐ VIMPAT ☐ DILANTIN ☐ DEPAKOTE

☐ LAMICTAL ☐ OTHER: _____

START DATE: _____

END DATE: _____

DOSE: _____

NOTES: _____

_____

_____

NAME OF MEDICATION: _____

☐ KEPPRA ☐ VIMPAT ☐ DILANTIN ☐ DEPAKOTE

☐ LAMICTAL ☐ OTHER: _____

START DATE: _____

END DATE: _____

DOSE: _____

NOTES: _____

_____

_____

NAME OF MEDICATION: _____

☐ KEPPRA   ☐ VIMPAT   ☐ DILANTIN   ☐ DEPAKOTE

☐ LAMICTAL   ☐ OTHER: _____

START DATE: _____

END DATE: _____

DOSE: _____

NOTES: _____

_____

_____

_____

NAME OF MEDICATION: _____

☐ KEPPRA   ☐ VIMPAT   ☐ DILANTIN   ☐ DEPAKOTE

☐ LAMICTAL   ☐ OTHER: _____

START DATE: _____

END DATE: _____

DOSE: _____

NOTES: _____

_____

_____

NAME OF MEDICATION:

☐ KEPPRA ☐ VIMPAT ☐ DILANTIN ☐ DEPAKOTE

☐ LAMICTAL ☐ OTHER: _____

START DATE:

END DATE:

DOSE:

NOTES:

NAME OF MEDICATION:

☐ KEPPRA ☐ VIMPAT ☐ DILANTIN ☐ DEPAKOTE

☐ LAMICTAL ☐ OTHER: _____

START DATE:

END DATE:

DOSE:

NOTES:

NAME OF MEDICATION:

☐ KEPPRA   ☐ VIMPAT   ☐ DILANTIN   ☐ DEPAKOTE

☐ LAMICTAL   ☐ OTHER: _____

START DATE:

END DATE:

DOSE:

NOTES:

NAME OF MEDICATION:

☐ KEPPRA   ☐ VIMPAT   ☐ DILANTIN   ☐ DEPAKOTE

☐ LAMICTAL   ☐ OTHER: _____

START DATE:

END DATE:

DOSE:

NOTES:

LOMUSTINE MEDICATION LOG

START DATE (42 DAY CYCLE): _____

END DATE: _____

DOSE: _____

NOTES: _____

_____

_____

_____

START DATE (42 DAY CYCLE): _____

END DATE: _____

DOSE: _____

NOTES: _____

_____

_____

_____

START DATE (42 DAY CYCLE): _____

END DATE: _____

DOSE: _____

NOTES: _____

_____

_____

START DATE (42 DAY CYCLE):

END DATE:

DOSE:

NOTES:

START DATE (42 DAY CYCLE):

END DATE:

DOSE:

NOTES:

START DATE (42 DAY CYCLE):

END DATE:

DOSE:

NOTES:

START DATE (42 DAY CYCLE):

END DATE:

DOSE:

NOTES:

START DATE (42 DAY CYCLE):

END DATE:

DOSE:

NOTES:

START DATE (42 DAY CYCLE):

END DATE:

DOSE:

NOTES:

START DATE (42 DAY CYCLE): _____

END DATE: _____

DOSE: _____

NOTES: _____

_____

_____

_____

START DATE (42 DAY CYCLE): _____

END DATE: _____

DOSE: _____

NOTES: _____

_____

_____

_____

START DATE (42 DAY CYCLE): _____

END DATE: _____

DOSE: _____

NOTES: _____

_____

_____

_____

AVASTIN MEDICATION LOG

START DATE (14 DAY CYCLE):

END DATE:

DOSE:

INFUSION CENTER:

NOTES:

START DATE (14 DAY CYCLE):

END DATE:

DOSE:

INFUSION CENTER:

NOTES:

START DATE (14 DAY CYCLE):

END DATE:

DOSE:

INFUSION CENTER:

NOTES:

START DATE (14 DAY CYCLE): _____

END DATE: _____

DOSE: _____

INFUSION CENTER: _____

NOTES: _____

_____

START DATE (14 DAY CYCLE): _____

END DATE: _____

DOSE: _____

INFUSION CENTER: _____

NOTES: _____

_____

START DATE (14 DAY CYCLE): _____

END DATE: _____

DOSE: _____

INFUSION CENTER: _____

NOTES: _____

_____

START DATE (14 DAY CYCLE):

END DATE:

DOSE:

INFUSION CENTER:

NOTES:

START DATE (14 DAY CYCLE):

END DATE:

DOSE:

INFUSION CENTER:

NOTES:

START DATE (14 DAY CYCLE):

END DATE:

DOSE:

INFUSION CENTER:

NOTES:

START DATE (14 DAY CYCLE):

END DATE:

DOSE:

INFUSION CENTER:

NOTES:

START DATE (14 DAY CYCLE):

END DATE:

DOSE:

INFUSION CENTER:

NOTES:

START DATE (14 DAY CYCLE):

END DATE:

DOSE:

INFUSION CENTER:

NOTES:

START DATE (14 DAY CYCLE):

END DATE:

DOSE:

INFUSION CENTER:

NOTES:

START DATE (14 DAY CYCLE):

END DATE:

DOSE:

INFUSION CENTER:

NOTES:

START DATE (14 DAY CYCLE):

END DATE:

DOSE:

INFUSION CENTER:

NOTES:

START DATE (14 DAY CYCLE):

END DATE:

DOSE:

INFUSION CENTER:

NOTES:

START DATE (14 DAY CYCLE):

END DATE:

DOSE:

INFUSION CENTER:

NOTES:

START DATE (14 DAY CYCLE):

END DATE:

DOSE:

INFUSION CENTER:

NOTES:

START DATE (14 DAY CYCLE):

END DATE:

DOSE:

INFUSION CENTER:

NOTES:

START DATE (14 DAY CYCLE):

END DATE:

DOSE:

INFUSION CENTER:

NOTES:

START DATE (14 DAY CYCLE):

END DATE:

DOSE:

INFUSION CENTER:

NOTES:

START DATE (14 DAY CYCLE):

END DATE:

DOSE:

INFUSION CENTER:

NOTES:

START DATE (14 DAY CYCLE):

END DATE:

DOSE:

INFUSION CENTER:

NOTES:

START DATE (14 DAY CYCLE):

END DATE:

DOSE:

INFUSION CENTER:

NOTES:

OTHER MEDICATION LOG

MEDICATION NAME:

REASON:

START DATE:

END DATE:

DOSE:

NOTES:

MEDICATION NAME:

REASON:

START DATE:

END DATE:

DOSE:

NOTES:

MEDICATION NAME:

REASON:

START DATE:

END DATE:

DOSE:

NOTES:

MEDICATION NAME:

REASON:

START DATE:

END DATE:

DOSE:

NOTES:

MEDICATION NAME:

REASON:

START DATE:

END DATE:

DOSE:

NOTES:

MEDICATION NAME:

REASON:

START DATE:

END DATE:

DOSE:

NOTES:

MEDICATION NAME:
_____

REASON:
_____

START DATE:
_____

END DATE:
_____

DOSE:
_____

_____

NOTES:
_____

_____

_____

MEDICATION NAME:
_____

REASON:
_____

START DATE:
_____

END DATE:
_____

DOSE:
_____

_____

NOTES:
_____

_____

MEDICATION NAME:

REASON:

START DATE:

END DATE:

DOSE:

NOTES:

MEDICATION NAME:

REASON:

START DATE:

END DATE:

DOSE:

NOTES:

NOTES

NOTES

CALENDAR

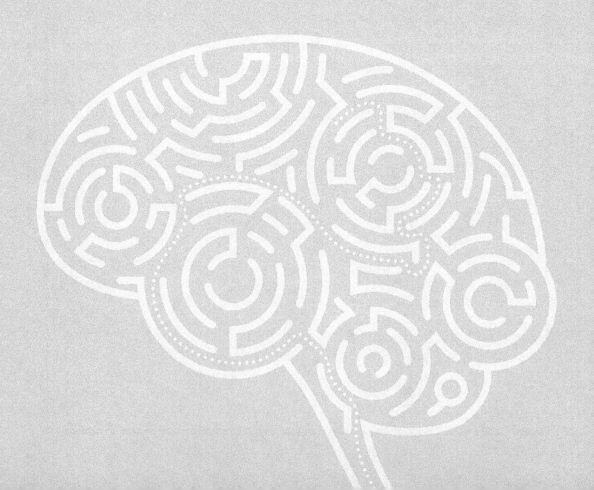

MON. DATE:	**TUES.** DATE:	**WED.** DATE:
THURS. DATE:	**FRI.** DATE:	**SAT.** DATE:
		SUN. DATE:

MON. DATE:	**TUES.** DATE:	**WED.** DATE:
THURS. DATE:	**FRI.** DATE:	**SAT.** DATE:
		SUN. DATE:

MON. DATE:	**TUES.** DATE:	**WED.** DATE:

THURS. DATE:	**FRI.** DATE:	**SAT.** DATE:
		SUN. DATE:

MON. DATE:	**TUES.** DATE:	**WED.** DATE:

THURS. DATE:	**FRI.** DATE:	**SAT.** DATE:
		SUN. DATE:

MON. DATE:	TUES. DATE:	WED. DATE:

THURS. DATE:	FRI. DATE:	SAT. DATE:
		SUN. DATE:

MON. DATE:	TUES. DATE:	WED. DATE:

THURS. DATE:	FRI. DATE:	SAT. DATE:
		SUN. DATE:

MON. DATE:	TUES. DATE:	WED. DATE:
THURS. DATE:	FRI. DATE:	SAT. DATE:
		SUN. DATE:

MON. DATE:	TUES. DATE:	WED. DATE:
THURS. DATE:	FRI. DATE:	SAT. DATE:
		SUN. DATE:

MON. DATE:	TUES. DATE:	WED. DATE:
THURS. DATE:	**FRI.** DATE:	**SAT.** DATE:
		SUN. DATE:

MON. DATE:	TUES. DATE:	WED. DATE:
THURS. DATE:	**FRI.** DATE:	**SAT.** DATE:
		SUN. DATE:

MON. DATE:	TUES. DATE:	WED. DATE:

THURS. DATE:	FRI. DATE:	SAT. DATE:
		SUN. DATE:

MON. DATE:	TUES. DATE:	WED. DATE:

THURS. DATE:	FRI. DATE:	SAT. DATE:
		SUN. DATE:

MON. DATE:	TUES. DATE:	WED. DATE:
THURS. DATE:	FRI. DATE:	SAT. DATE:
		SUN. DATE:

MON. DATE:	TUES. DATE:	WED. DATE:
THURS. DATE:	FRI. DATE:	SAT. DATE:
		SUN. DATE:

MON. DATE:	**TUES.** DATE:	**WED.** DATE:
THURS. DATE:	**FRI.** DATE:	**SAT.** DATE:
		SUN. DATE:

MON. DATE:	**TUES.** DATE:	**WED.** DATE:
THURS. DATE:	**FRI.** DATE:	**SAT.** DATE:
		SUN. DATE:

MON. DATE:	**TUES.** DATE:	**WED.** DATE:

THURS. DATE:	**FRI.** DATE:	**SAT.** DATE:
		SUN. DATE:

MON. DATE:	**TUES.** DATE:	**WED.** DATE:

THURS. DATE:	**FRI.** DATE:	**SAT.** DATE:
		SUN. DATE:

MON. DATE:	TUES. DATE:	WED. DATE:
THURS. DATE:	FRI. DATE:	SAT. DATE:
		SUN. DATE:

MON. DATE:	TUES. DATE:	WED. DATE:
THURS. DATE:	FRI. DATE:	SAT. DATE:
		SUN. DATE:

MON. DATE:	TUES. DATE:	WED. DATE:
THURS. DATE:	FRI. DATE:	SAT. DATE:
		SUN. DATE:

MON. DATE:	TUES. DATE:	WED. DATE:
THURS. DATE:	FRI. DATE:	SAT. DATE:
		SUN. DATE:

MON. DATE:	**TUES.** DATE:	**WED.** DATE:

THURS. DATE:	**FRI.** DATE:	**SAT.** DATE:
		SUN. DATE:

MON. DATE:	**TUES.** DATE:	**WED.** DATE:

THURS. DATE:	**FRI.** DATE:	**SAT.** DATE:
		SUN. DATE:

NOTES

NOTES

NOTES

NOTES

NOTES

NOTES

NOTES

NOTES

NOTES

CONTACT US

WWW.DRTHOMASGRUBER.COM

Printed in the USA
CPSIA information can be obtained
at www.ICGtesting.com
JSHW052001150824
68134JS00059B/2587

9 781642 254105